PALEO FOR FOOD LOVERS

GLUTEN FREE AND GRAIN FREE COOKBOOK

Disclaimer

What You Will Find In This Book?

Life has become so busy these days that we don't even get time to take care of our health. We eat whatever we get our hands on, without thinking for a moment how healthy or unhealthy it is. Paleo diet is the perfect solution for all such people. It is healthy and very easy to follow.

Paleo fully read as Paleolithic, is a diet based on wild plants and animals that were consumed in the cavemen era. The fact that this diet belongs to the ancient Paleolithic era does not imply that it is tasteless and difficult to follow. On the contrary, it is very easy to make Paleo food. The best part is that there is a Paleo recipe for every meal and taste preference.

If you want to try out this diet, this book is the perfect guide for you. It contains the following:

1. 50 Paleo recipes for all mealtimes

2. Recipes for breakfast, appetizers, dips, main course, dessert and much more…

3. Cooking time and serving size of each recipe.

4. Nutritional facts of each recipe so that you can manage your calories accordingly

Paleo does not restrict you to eat your favorite food. Whether it is pizza, steak, cake or cookies, there is a Paleo recipe for everything. You just have to find it and you can eat anything you want, but in Paleo style.

So don't just stop here. Go ahead and try out a few. You are surely going to fall in love with the Paleo diet.

Contents

Disclaimer 2

What You Will Find In This Book? 3

Paleo Breakfast Recipes 13

    Sweet Potato and Pepper Casserole 13

        Serving Size 13

        Cooking Time 13

        Nutritional Facts (Values per Serving) 13

        Ingredients 13

        Preparation Method 13

    Paleo Friendly Breakfast Platter 15

        Serving Size 15

        Cooking Time 15

        Nutritional Facts (Values per Serving) 15

        Ingredients 15

        Preparation Method 15

    Shredded Pork Casserole 17

        Serving Size 17

        Cooking Time 17

        Nutritional Facts (Values per Serving) 17

        Ingredients 17

        Preparation Method 17

    Ham and Egg Muffins 19

        Serving Size 19

        Cooking Time 19

        Nutritional Facts (Values per Serving) 19

        Ingredients 19

        Preparation Method 19

    Coconut Mushroom Quiche 21

        Serving Size 21

        Cooking Time 21

        Nutritional Facts (Values per Serving) 21

        Ingredients 21

        Preparation Method 21

Fruit Yogurt Crumble 23

    Serving Size 23

    Cooking Time 23

    Nutritional Facts (Values per Serving)..................................... 23

    Ingredients 23

    Preparation Method.. 23

Almond Milk Muffins.. 24

    Serving Size 24

    Cooking Time 24

    Nutritional Facts (Values per Serving)..................................... 24

    Ingredients 24

    Preparation Method.. 24

Paleo Style Breakfast Patties 26

    Serving Size 26

    Cooking Time 26

    Nutritional Facts (Values per Serving)..................................... 26

    Ingredients 26

    Preparation Method.. 26

Sweet Potato and Agave Pancakes... 28

    Serving Size 28

    Cooking Time 28

    Nutritional Facts (Values per Pancake)................................... 28

    Ingredients 28

    Preparation Method.. 28

Paleo Appetizer Recipes 30

  Tex Mex Salad 30

    Serving Size 30

    Cooking Time 30

    Nutritional Facts (Values per Serving)..................................... 30

    Ingredients 30

    Preparation Method.. 31

  Kale Krisps 32

    Serving Size 32

    Cooking Time 32

Nutritional Facts (Values per Serving)..32

Ingredients 32

Preparation Method...32

Tuna Steak Salad 34

Serving Size 34

Cooking Time 34

Nutritional Facts (Values per Serving)..34

Ingredients 34

Preparation Method...34

Guacamole Fajita Salad 36

Serving Size 36

Cooking Time 36

Nutritional Facts (Values per Serving)..36

Ingredients 36

Preparation Method...36

Jalapeno Salad 38

Serving Size 38

Cooking Time 38

Nutritional Facts (Values per Serving)..38

Ingredients 38

Preparation Method...38

Pineapple and Tuna Crumble 40

Serving Size 40

Cooking Time 40

Nutritional Facts (Values per Serving)..40

Ingredients 40

Preparation Method...40

Shallot Fried Sprouts 42

Serving Size 42

Cooking Time 42

Nutritional Facts (Values per Serving)..42

Ingredients 42

Preparation Method...42

Smoky Squash Salad 44

Serving Size 44

Cooking Time 44

Nutritional Facts (Values per Serving) 44

Ingredients 44

Preparation Method 44

Mock Caesar Salad – Paleo Style 45

Serving Size 45

Cooking Time 45

Nutritional Facts (Values per Serving) 45

Ingredients 45

Preparation Method 45

Paleo Style Honey Crepes 47

Serving Size 47

Cooking Time 47

Nutritional Facts (Values per Serving) 47

Ingredients 47

Preparation Method 47

Mango and Jalapeno Salad 48

Serving Size 48

Cooking Time 48

Nutritional Facts (Values per Serving) 48

Ingredients 48

Preparation Method 48

Jicama and Snow Peas Salad 50

Serving Size 50

Cooking Time 50

Nutritional Facts (Values per Serving) 50

Ingredients 50

Preparation Method 50

Paleo Dips Recipes 52

Paleo Adobo Dip 52

Serving Size 52

Cooking Time 52

Nutritional Facts (Values per Serving) 52

Ingredients 52

Preparation Method 52

Mustard Lemon Dip 53

Serving Size 53

Cooking Time 53

Nutritional Facts (Values per Serving)... 53

Ingredients 53

Preparation Method 53

Zucchini Hummus 55

Serving Size 55

Cooking Time 55

Nutritional Facts (Values per Serving)... 55

Ingredients 55

Preparation Method 55

Paleo Style Habanero Salsa 57

Serving Size 57

Cooking Time 57

Nutritional Facts (Values per Serving)... 57

Ingredients 57

Preparation Method 57

BBQ Flavored Spicy Sauce 58

Serving Size 58

Cooking Time 58

Nutritional Facts (Values per Serving)... 58

Ingredients 58

Preparation Method 59

Roasted Red Walnut Dip 60

Serving Size 60

Cooking Time 60

Nutritional Facts (Values per Serving)... 60

Ingredients 60

Preparation Method 60

Hot and Fiery Sauce 62

Serving Size 62

Cooking Time 62

Nutritional Facts (Values per Serving) 62

Ingredients 62

Preparation Method 62

Paleo Main Course Recipes 64

Wild Salmon Delight 64

Serving Size 64

Cooking Time 64

Nutritional Facts (Values per Serving) 64

Ingredients 64

Preparation Method 64

Paleo Beef with Juicy Butternut Squash 66

Serving Size 66

Cooking Time 66

Nutritional Facts (Values per Serving) 66

Ingredients 66

Preparation Method 67

Spaghetti Squash with Veggie Fry 68

Serving Size 68

Cooking Time 68

Nutritional Facts (Values per Serving) 68

Ingredients 68

Preparation Method 69

Pork Lime Strips 70

Serving Size 70

Cooking Time 70

Nutritional Facts (Values per Serving) 70

Ingredients 70

Preparation Method 70

Taco Stuffed Peppers 72

Serving Size 72

Cooking Time 72

Nutritional Facts (Values per Serving) 72

Ingredients 72

Preparation Method 72

Shrimp and Chicken Jambalaya 74

Serving Size 74

Cooking Time 74

Nutritional Facts (Values per Serving) 74

Ingredients 74

Preparation Method 75

Cheesy Bacon Rolls 76

Serving Size 76

Cooking Time 76

Nutritional Facts (Values per Serving) 76

Ingredients 76

Preparation Method 76

Spicy Pork Chops with Grilled Vegetables 78

Serving Size 78

Cooking Time 78

Nutritional Facts (Values per Serving) 78

Ingredients 78

Preparation Method 78

Paleo Friendly Cheesy Beef Pizza 80

Serving Size 80

Cooking Time 80

Nutritional Facts (Values per Serving) 80

Ingredients 80

Preparation Method 81

Spicy Turkey Meatballs 82

Serving Size 82

Cooking Time 82

Nutritional Facts (Values per Serving) 82

Ingredients 82

Preparation Method 82

Lemon Shrimp Delight 84

Serving Size 84

Cooking Time 84

Nutritional Facts (Values per Serving)..84

Ingredients 84

Preparation Method..84

Almond Tuna Patties 86

Serving Size 86

Cooking Time..86

Nutritional Facts (Values per Serving)..86

Ingredients 86

Preparation Method..86

Paleo Dessert Recipes...88

Avocado Chocolate Mousse 88

Serving Size 88

Cooking Time..88

Nutritional Facts (Values per Serving)..88

Ingredients 88

Preparation Method..88

Apple and Pear Cake with Honey Walnut Topping 90

Serving Size 90

Cooking Time..90

Nutritional Facts (Values per Serving)..90

Ingredients for Cake..90

Ingredients for Honey Walnut Topping...91

Preparation Method..91

Zesty Date Tarts 93

Serving Size 93

Cooking Time..93

Nutritional Facts (Values per Tart) 93

Ingredients for Crust...93

Ingredients for Filling..93

Preparation Method..93

Chocolicious Banana Cinnamon Loaf...95

Serving Size 95

Cooking Time..95

Nutritional Facts (Values per Serving)..95

Ingredients 95

Preparation Method.. 95

Paleo Style Pumpkin Vanilla Custard 97

  Serving Size 97

  Cooking Time 97

  Nutritional Facts (Values per Serving).. 97

  Ingredients 97

  Preparation Method.. 97

Cranberry and Nut Protein Bars 99

  Serving Size 99

  Cooking Time 99

  Nutritional Facts (Values per Serving).. 99

  Ingredients 99

  Preparation Method.. 100

Applesauce Muffins with Raspberry Topping..................................... 101

  Serving Size 101

  Cooking Time 101

  Nutritional Facts (Values per Serving).. 101

  Ingredients 101

  Preparation Method.. 101

Frozen Fruit Delight 103

  Serving Size 103

  Cooking Time 103

  Nutritional Facts (Values per Serving).. 103

  Ingredients 103

  Preparation Method.. 103

Banana Coconut Waffles 104

  Serving Size 104

  Cooking Time 104

  Nutritional Facts (Values per Serving).. 104

  Ingredients 104

  Preparation Method.. 105

Paleo Breakfast Recipes

Sweet Potato and Pepper Casserole

Serving Size

Serves 6

Cooking Time

Approx. 60 minutes

Nutritional Facts (Values per Serving)

Calories: 525

Total Carbohydrate: 28 g

Cholesterol: 250 mg

Protein: 22 g

Total Fat: 37.6 g

Ingredients

¾ cup coconut milk

1 ½ pounds sweet potatoes, peeled and shredded

1 medium sized onion, chopped

1 roasted red bell pepper, peeled, seeded and diced

8 oz. white mushrooms, cut into slices

6 eggs

1 pound Italian sausage

¾ tsp ground black pepper, divided

2 Tbsp lard

1 ½ tsp kosher salt, divided

Preparation Method

Set oven to preheat at 375ºF.

Grease a casserole baking dish with lard.

Soak the shredded sweet potatoes in ice water. Set aside.

Crumble the sausages in a skillet. Cook over medium heat till the sausage is no longer pink.

Line a bowl with paper towel and put the cooked crumbled sausage in it. Set aside.

Add mushrooms in the same skillet.

Reduce the heat to medium and cook mushrooms till they are brown and crispy. Do not overcrowd the skillet with mushrooms. Cook in batches if necessary.

Remove the mushrooms with a slotted spoon and add them to the crumbled sausage.

Now put onions in the same skillet. Add ½ tsp more lard, if necessary.

Sauté for 4 – 5 minutes, till the onions are tender and golden.

Add the sautéed onions to the mushroom-sausage mixture.

Stir in the roasted chopped bell pepper. Mix well and set aside.

Drain the shredded potatoes and place them on a few layers of power towel. Pat dry.

Season the sweet potatoes with 1 teaspoon salt and half teaspoon ground black pepper. Set aside.

Whisk the eggs in a large bowl along with coconut milk and the remaining salt and pepper.

Spread the seasoned sweet potatoes in the bottom of the greased baking dish.

Spread the sausage mixture over the sweet potatoes, followed by the egg mixture.

Cover the baking dish with foil and put it in the oven for 20 – 30 minutes or until a toothpick when inserted in the center of the casserole comes out clean.

Remove the foil and bake uncovered for 5 – 10 more minutes, till it is lightly brown on the top.

Let it cool on the rack for 10 minutes.

Serve!

Paleo Friendly Breakfast Platter

Serving Size

Serves 2

Cooking Time

10 minutes

Nutritional Facts (Values per Serving)

Calories: 627

Total Carbohydrate: 8.2 g

Cholesterol: 466.5 mg

Protein: 29.4 g

Total Fat: 54.4 g

Ingredients

4 large eggs

4 Tbsp Coconut oil

1 ripe avocado, mashed

4 Tbsp White vinegar

Half cup leftover cooked chicken or beef, chopped or ground.

4 Tbsp mixed spices (turmeric, salt, coriander, smoked paprika, cumin, pepper)

Preparation Method

Fill a pot with about 4 inches of water.

Stir in the white vinegar. Bring it to boil over medium-high flame.

When the water is lightly boiling, reduce the heat to medium.

Crack the eggs into the water and poach them till the egg yolk starts to thicken. This should take about 3 minutes.

Take the eggs out and divided them equally onto two serving plates.

Place another nonstick pan on medium flame and heat the coconut oil in it.

When the oil is hot, add the leftover meat and spices to it. Stir to mix.

Now reduce the heat to low and stir for 2 minutes.

Take the meat out and divided them on the serving plates.

Finally, divide the mashed avocado equally on the two serving plates.

Lightly mix all the things on the serving plate and serve!

Shredded Pork Casserole

Serving Size

Serves 7 – 8

Cooking Time

40 minutes

Nutritional Facts (Values per Serving)

Calories: 210

Total Carbohydrate: 2.5 g

Cholesterol: 230 mg

Protein: 23.3 g

Total Fat: 11.4 g

Ingredients

1 Tbsp extra virgin olive oil

1 cup chopped zucchini

16 oz. shredded pork tenderloin

3 cloves of garlic, diced

2 Tbsp chopped basil

1 medium sized red onion, chopped

8 large eggs, scrambled

Dash of freshly ground black pepper

Dash of kosher salt

Lard, to grease the dish

Preparation Method

Set the oven to preheat at 350°F.

Grease a casserole baking dish with lard.

Put the oil in a skillet and combine the onions and garlic in it.

Sauté over medium-high heat till the onions are caramelized.

Remove the skillet off the heat.

Take a bowl and add in it the eggs, basil, zucchini, pork, salt and pepper. Whisk well,

Stir in the caramelized onion and garlic. Mix well.

Pour it in the greased baking dish.

Put it in the preheated oven for 30 minutes or till the center of the casserole is set.

Now place the dish under the broiler for 3 – 5 minutes, to brown the top of the casserole.

Cut it into sizeable portions and serve!

Ham and Egg Muffins

Serving Size

Makes 8 muffins

Cooking Time

20 minutes

Nutritional Facts (Values per Serving)

Calories: 308

Total Carbohydrate: 6.8 g

Cholesterol: 454 mg

Protein: 23.8 g

Total Fat: 20.5 g

Ingredients

2 Tbsp water

8 eggs

¼ tsp kosher salt

1 cup chopped onion

8 oz. cooked ham, crumbled

Pinch of ground black pepper

1 cup chopped red bell pepper

Preparation Method

Set the oven to preheat at 350°F.

Line a muffin pan with paper liners.

Beat all the eggs in the large bowl.

Stir in all the remaining ingredients. Mix well.

Pour the mixture into the paper-lined muffin cups, while filling ¾ of each cup.

Bake for 18 – 20 minutes, till the muffins are set in the center.

Enjoy!

Coconut Mushroom Quiche

Serving Size

Serves 6

Cooking Time

30 minutes

Nutritional Facts (Values per Serving)

Calories: 193.6

Total Carbohydrate: 3.7 g

Cholesterol: 370 mg

Protein: 13.4 g

Total Fat: 13.6 g

Ingredients

5 white mushrooms, cut into slices

15 large eggs

1 ½ tsp baking powder

3 cloves of garlic, minced

1 small onion, diced

Freshly ground black pepper to taste

1 ½ cup coconut milk

3 cups fresh chopped spinach

Sea salt to taste

Lard, to grease

Preparation Method

Set the oven to preheat at 350°F.

Grease a 9 x 11 baking dish with lard.

Beat the eggs in a large bowl along with the coconut milk. Whisk well.

Start adding in other ingredients while you are beating the eggs.

When all the ingredients are thoroughly whisked in the eggs, transfer the entire mixture to the greased dish,

Put it in the preheated oven for 40 minutes, or till it is set in the middle.

Cut into equal portions and serve!

Fruit Yogurt Crumble

Serving Size

Serves 6

Cooking Time

2 minutes

Nutritional Facts (Values per Serving)

Calories: 251

Total Carbohydrate: 46.7 g

Cholesterol: 3.3 mg

Protein: 8.4 g

Total Fat: 5.7 g

Ingredients

1 small container of plain Greek yogurt (fat free)

1 cup chopped raw celery

4 small apples, finely diced

¼ cup hulled sunflower seeds (salt-free)

Half cup raisins

Preparation Method

Combine all the ingredients in a serving bowl.

Serve immediately.

Almond Milk Muffins

Serving Size

Makes 12 muffins

Cooking Time

20 minutes

Nutritional Facts (Values per Serving)

Calories: 316.4

Total Carbohydrate: 21.3 g

Cholesterol: 93 mg

Protein: 8 g

Total Fat: 23.4 g

Ingredients

Half cup chocolate chips

1 cup almond flour

4 Tbsp honey

6 large eggs

1 tsp kosher salt

1 cup almond milk

Half cup melted coconut oil

Half cup coconut flour

Half cup chopped mixed nuts

1 tsp baking soda

Preparation Method

Set the oven to preheat at 350°F.

Line a muffin pan with paper liners.

Combine all the dry ingredients in a large bowl.

Add eggs to it. Mix well.

Stir in the coconut milk, honey and almond milk. Mix till the ingredients are thoroughly blended.

Pour the batter into the paper-lined muffin cups, while filling ¾ of each cup.

Bake for 18 – 20 minutes, or until a toothpick when inserted in the center comes out clean.

Enjoy!

Paleo Style Breakfast Patties

Serving Size

Serves 8

Cooking Time

15 – 20 minutes

Nutritional Facts (Values per Serving)

Calories: 118

Total Carbohydrate: 0.3 g

Cholesterol: 37 mg

Protein: 10.1 g

Total Fat: 8.2 g

Ingredients

1 lb. ground pork

¼ tsp cayenne pepper

1 tsp fresh thyme, finely chopped

¾ tsp freshly ground black pepper

¼ tsp red pepper flakes

¼ tsp chopped fresh rosemary

1 tsp kosher salt

2 tsp chopped fresh sage leaves

¼ tsp ground nutmeg

Preparation Method

Combine all the ingredients in a large bowl. Mix well.

Knead with hands so that all the spices are thoroughly incorporated in the pork.

Form the mixture into 8 patties.

Place the patties in a nonstick skillet over medium flame.

Cook till the patties are brown one side, about 10 minutes.

Flip and cook till the other side is brown and pork is fully cooked through, 6 – 8 minutes.

Serve with any of the Paleo dip.

Enjoy!

Sweet Potato and Agave Pancakes

Serving Size

Makes 10 – 12 pancakes

Cooking Time

15 minutes plus about 5 minutes per pancake

Nutritional Facts (Values per Pancake)

Calories: 127

Total Carbohydrate: 14 g

Cholesterol: 130 mg

Protein: 5 g

Total Fat: 5.7 g

Ingredients

3 medium sweet potatoes, peeled and cut into 1-inch cubes

6 free range eggs

1 tsp sea salt

2 tsp ground cinnamon, divided

1 granny smith apple, peeled and finely diced

1 tsp vanilla essence

1 Tbsp agave nectar

8 Tbsp coconut flour (about half cup)

2 Tbsp grass-fed butter

1 tsp of baking powder

Coconut oil to fry the pancakes

Preparation Method

Fill a large saucepan with water and add ½ tsp salt to it.

Bring it to a boil and then add the sweet potatoes to the boiling water.

Boil till the potatoes are soft, for about 15 minutes.

Drain and set aside.

Combine the butter and 1 teaspoon ground cinnamon in a skillet. Heat it over medium flame.

When the butter is melted and hot, add the diced apples to it.

Sauté the apples till softened. Set aside.

Take a small bowl and combine the coconut flour, baking powder, sea salt and the remaining cinnamon. Mix well.

Place the sweet potatoes in a food processor.

Pulse till it becomes a smooth puree.

Add the vanilla extract, agave nectar and eggs to the processor. Pulse till the ingredients are thoroughly mixed.

Finally, add the coconut flour mixture to the processor. Pulse to mix.

Now heat a griddle and put a dab of coconut oil in it.

Scoop about one cup of batter to make the pancake.

Fry individual pancakes on medium-low heat. Flip when one side is brown.

Top up the pancakes with the apple mixture. Enjoy!

Paleo Appetizer Recipes

Tex Mex Salad

Serving Size

Serves 8

Cooking Time

15 – 20 minutes

Nutritional Facts (Values per Serving)

Calories: 385

Total Carbohydrate: 18.5 g

Cholesterol: 83 mg

Protein: 25 g

Total Fat: 24.7 g

Ingredients

2 onions, diced

4 Romaine hearts, finely chopped

6 cups cherry tomatoes, halved

4 cloves of garlic, crushed

4 Tbsp red chili powder

1 tsp cayenne pepper

2 Tbsp fresh lime juice

Half cup sour cream

4 tsp ground cumin

Half cup grated cheddar cheese

2 pounds ground beef

4 tsp garlic powder

Ground black pepper to taste

2/3 cup fresh chopped cilantro

1 cup salsa sauce (Paleo friendly)

Sea salt to taste

Preparation Method

Take a bowl and add in the chili powder, cumin, salt, garlic powder, cayenne pepper and ground black pepper. Mix well and set aside.

Place a nonstick pan over medium flame.

Cook meat in it till it is brown.

Add onion and garlic to the meat.

Sauté till the onion is translucent.

Add the spice mixture.

Cook and stir for 3 more minutes.

Take another bowl and combine the sour cream, salsa and lime juice in it. Mix well.

Spread the romaine lettuce onto one large serving plate (you can also make 8 individual servings).

Scoop the cooked meat over the lettuce.

Top it up with the salsa mixture, followed by cherry tomatoes, cheese and cilantro.

Serve!

Kale Krisps

Serving Size

Serves 7 – 8

Cooking Time

10 – 12 minutes

Nutritional Facts (Values per Serving)

Calories: 110

Total Carbohydrate: 16 g

Cholesterol: 0.1 mg

Protein: 5.1 g

Total Fat: 5 g

Ingredients

2 large bunches of Kale, pat dry and stems removed

2 Tbsp extra virgin olive oil

Ground black pepper to taste

Sea salt to taste

Preparation Method

Preheat the oven to 400oF.

Tear the kale into large pieces.

Gather all the kale pieces in large bowl.

Season with olive oil, salt and pepper.

Use your hands so that all the ingredients are thoroughly coated.

Spread the seasoned kale pieces on a baking sheet.

Make sure the kale pieces do not overlap and the baking sheet is not over crowded with them. Bake in two batches if necessary.

Put it in the preheated oven for 10 – 12 minutes or until the leaves are crispy.

Serve with any of the Paleo Dips.

Tuna Steak Salad

Serving Size

Serves 7 – 8

Cooking Time

10 minutes

Nutritional Facts (Values per Serving)

Calories: 208

Total Carbohydrate: 18.5 g

Cholesterol: 44 mg

Protein: 29 g

Total Fat: 4 g

Ingredients

2 cups small watercress sprigs

2 lbs. (1-inch thick) tuna steaks, cut into four chunks

2 Tbsp – olive oil

2 tsp crystallized ginger

1 tsp ground coriander

½ tsp cayenne pepper

6 medium oranges, peeled and white piths removed

2 Tbsp rice vinegar

1 tsp kosher salt, divided

1 tsp ground aniseed, divided

½ tsp pepper

Preparation Method

Adjust the oven rack at least 5 inches above the broiler and set it to preheat at high.

Take a broiler pan and line it with aluminum foil.

In a bowl, combine the oranges, oil, rice vinegar, cayenne pepper, ground coriander, half of the ground aniseed, ginger and half of the salt. Mix well.

Stir in the watercress sprigs. Set aside.

Drizzle the tuna steak with pepper, remaining salt and the remaining aniseed.

Place the seasoned tuna steaks on the prepared broiler pan.

Broil the steak on medium heat, for 4 minutes on each side.

Transfer the broiled steak to the serving plate.

Top it up with orange-vinegar salad.

Enjoy!

Guacamole Fajita Salad

Serving Size

Serves 2

Cooking Time

25 – 30 minutes

Nutritional Facts (Values per Serving)

Calories: 806

Total Carbohydrate: 41 g

Cholesterol: 128 mg

Protein: 60.6 g

Total Fat: 46.6 g

Ingredients

16 ounces chicken breast (boneless and skinless)

2 red bell peppers, cut into slices

8 Tbsp salsa

2 Tbsp olive oil

1 medium sized onion, cut into slices

16 Tbsp guacamole

4 Tbsp fresh cilantro

4 cups shredded Romaine

Sea salt to taste

Freshly ground black pepper to taste

Preparation Method

Heat up a cast iron skillet.

Add olive oil to it.

Season the chicken breast with salt and pepper.

Cook it in the olive oil.

Transfer the chicken to a plate. Set aside.

Now put onion and bell peppers to the same skillet.

Cook over medium-high flame till the veggies are tender yet crispy, and the pepper strips are slightly charred. Turn off the heat.

When the chicken is cool enough to handle, cut it into strips.

Stir in the veggies.

To serve the salad, divide the chicken-veggie mixture equally on two serving plates.

Top up each serving with equal portions of romaine, salsa, guacamole and cilantro.

Enjoy!

Jalapeno Salad

Serving Size

Serves 6

Cooking Time

5 minutes

Nutritional Facts (Values per Serving)

Calories: 118

Total Carbohydrate: 8.2 g

Cholesterol: 0 mg

Protein: 1.7 g

Total Fat: 9.9 g

Ingredients

1 Italian plum tomato, diced

1 Tbsp fresh lime juice

2 ripe avocados, peeled and pitted

1 Tbsp chopped fresh cilantro

1 clove of garlic, crushed

Half cup minced onion

Salt to taste

1 Jalapeno pepper, diced

Freshly ground black pepper to taste

Preparation Method

Place the avocados in a bowl.

Pour the lime juice over it.

Coarsely mash the avocados with a fork.

Stir in all the other ingredients.

Serve!

Pineapple and Tuna Crumble

Serving Size

Serves 6

Cooking Time

About 60 minutes

Nutritional Facts (Values per Serving)

Calories: 458

Total Carbohydrate: 48.7 g

Cholesterol: 87 mg

Protein: 33.2 g

Total Fat: 16 g

Ingredients

1½ cup almond flour

Half cup almond milk

2 free range eggs

12 oz. tuna (home cooked or canned)

1 cup coconut flour

Half cup orange juice

2 Tbsp baking powder

4 Tbsp extra virgin olive oil

2 cups chopped pineapple

Preparation Method

Except for olive oil, combine all the other ingredients in a large bowl.

Whisk till it becomes a smooth lump-free batter.

Place a nonstick skillet over medium flame and heat oil in it.

When the oil is hot, pour a scoopful of the batter in it.

Cook for 3 minutes, flip over and cook for another 3 minutes. Likewise cook for a total of 15 minutes, while flipping over the patty after every 3 minutes, till the patty is crispy.

Repeat the same to make other patties.

Serve with any of the Paleo dips.

Shallot Fried Sprouts

Serving Size

Serves 7 – 8

Cooking Time

25 – 30 minutes

Nutritional Facts (Values per Serving)

Calories: 88

Total Carbohydrate: 11 g

Cholesterol: 0.2 mg

Protein: 4 g

Total Fat: 4.2 g

Ingredients

2 lbs. Brussels sprouts, trimmed

½ tsp freshly ground pepper

2 Tbsp extra virgin olive oil

½ tsp kosher salt

4 shallots, cut into slices

1 tsp dried thyme

2 cups vegetable broth

Preparation Method

Place a nonstick skillet over medium flame and heat oil in it.

When the oil it hot, add shallots and sprouts to the oil. Sauté till both the things starts to brown.

When the shallots and sprouts began to brown, stir in the salt, pepper, thyme and broth.

Reduce the flame to low.

Cover the pan and let it cook for 10 – 15 minutes, till the sprouts are tender.

Smoky Squash Salad

Serving Size

Serves 4

Cooking Time

5 minutes

Nutritional Facts (Values per Serving)

Calories: 467

Total Carbohydrate: 34 g

Cholesterol: 62.5 mg

Protein: 13.4 g

Total Fat: 33 g

Ingredients

1 cup chopped red pepper

1 spaghetti squash, cooked

1 cup diced tomatoes

4 Tbsp chopped red onion

Half cup coconut oil mayo

12 oz. smoked sausage, diced

Preparation Method

Combine all the ingredients in a large serving bowl.

Serve!

Mock Caesar Salad – Paleo Style

Serving Size

Serves 4

Cooking Time

5 minutes

Nutritional Facts (Values per Serving)

Calories: 168

Total Carbohydrate: 11 g

Cholesterol: 0.1 mg

Protein: 6.6 g

Total Fat: 12.5 g

Ingredients

2 ripe avocados

Half cup hemp seeds

6 Tbsp fresh lime juice

4 Tbsp water

6 cloves of garlic, crushed

2 Tbsp caper brine

4 Tbsp capers

4 tsp Dijon mustard

8 cups coarsely chopped romaine leaves

Sea salt to taste

Freshly ground black pepper to taste

Preparation Method

Except for hemp seeds and romaine leaves, combine all the other ingredients in a food processor.

Pulse till pureed.

Now take 4 serving plates and spread 2 cups of romaine leaves on each plate.

Pour equal portions of the puree on each serving of romaine.

Sprinkle hemp seeds and serve!

Paleo Style Honey Crepes

Serving Size

Makes 6 crepes (about 3 servings)

Cooking Time

25 – 30 minutes

Nutritional Facts (Values per Serving)

Calories: 118

Total Carbohydrate: 5.1 g

Cholesterol: 180 mg

Protein: 9 g

Total Fat: 7.2 g

Ingredients

2 tsp grass fed butter

2 tsp honey

5 eggs

Pinch of kosher salt

Half cup almond flour

Preparation Method

Take a large bowl and combine eggs, flour, honey and salt in it. Mix well.

Divide this mixture into six equal portions. Roll a ball of each portion.

Press each ball to make a crepe. You can also a rolling pin to do this.

Place a nonstick pan over medium flame and heat butter in it.

One by one cook all the crepes in the pan. Cook each crepe for 2 minutes on each side, or till is light brown.

Serve it with fresh strawberries and Paleo friendly maple syrup.

Mango and Jalapeno Salad

Serving Size

Serves 6

Cooking Time

15 minutes

Nutritional Facts (Values per Serving)

Calories: 268.7

Total Carbohydrate: 6.2 g

Cholesterol: 95 mg

Protein: 41.6 g

Total Fat: 8.5 g

Ingredients

6 cups cooked diced chicken

10 bacon strips, diced

2 cups diced mango

2 jalapeno peppers, seeded and finely diced

6 – 8 cups of shredded romaine leaves

1 cup Coconut oil mayo

1 cup diced red bell pepper

Chipotle powder to taste

Sliced almonds to garnish

Preparation Method

Combine the mayo and chipotle. Set aside.

Brown the bacon in a nonstick skillet, till it is slightly crispy.

Stir in the red pepper and jalapeno. Sauté till the peppers are tender and the bacon is completely crispy.

Stir in the cooked chicken. Stir to combine and cook till the chicken is heated through.

Finally, add the diced mango to the skillet. Cook for 2 more minutes.

Spread a handful of romaine on each serving plate.

Spoon a scoopful of the chicken-bacon mixture over the romaine in each plate.

Drizzle each serving with chipotle mayo.

Garnish with sliced almonds and serve!

Jicama and Snow Peas Salad

Serving Size

Serves 7 – 8

Cooking Time

5 – 10 minutes

Nutritional Facts (Values per Serving)

Calories: 138

Total Carbohydrate: 17 g

Cholesterol: 0.2 mg

Protein: 3 g

Total Fat: 7 g

Ingredients

6 Tbsp fresh orange juice

2 small jicama, peel and cut into thin strips

2 tsp – sugar

2 Tbsp white wine vinegar

2 Tbsp minced shallot

4 oranges, peeled and white piths removed

8 oz. snow peas, trimmed

4 Tbsp extra virgin olive oil

½ tsp kosher salt

Preparation Method

First, you need to fix a steamer basket in a saucepan.

Fill it with water up to 1 inch. Bring the water to boil.

When the water starts to boil, add the snow peas to it.

Steam the peas for 3 – 5 minutes, till the peas are soft.

Drain the water and transfer the peas in a bowl filled with ice cold water. Let rest for a while then drain.

Now take a large bowl and combine the orange juice, shallot, oil, salt, vinegar and sugar in it. Mix well.

Carefully remove the membranes of all the orange slices.

Discard the membranes and add the orange slices to the shallot-vinegar mixture. Mix well.

Finally, stir in the snow peas and jicama.

Enjoy!

Paleo Dips Recipes

Paleo Adobo Dip

Serving Size

Serves 16

Cooking Time

5 minutes

Nutritional Facts (Values per Serving)

Calories: 133

Total Carbohydrate: 1.3 g

Cholesterol: 5 mg

Protein: 0.2 g

Total Fat: 0.2 g

Ingredients

1 cup chopped fresh cilantro

4 Chipotle peppers in adobo sauce

1 cup Paleo friendly Mayonnaise

2 cloves of garlic

2 Tbsp fresh lime juice

4 Tbsp extra virgin olive oil

Preparation Method

Combine all the ingredients in a food processor.

Pulse till it becomes a smooth puree.

Enjoy!

Mustard Lemon Dip

Serving Size

Serves 15

Cooking Time

10 – 15 minutes

Nutritional Facts (Values per Serving)

Calories: 125

Total Carbohydrate: 0.2 g

Cholesterol: 13 mg

Protein: 0.4 g

Total Fat: 13.9 g

Ingredients

½ cup avocado oil

1 ½ Tbsp fresh lemon juice

1 egg

½ tsp mustard powder

¼ tsp white pepper

½ cup olive oil

Preparation Method

Crack the egg in a food processor.

Now add the mustard powder and lemon juice to the processor.

Cover the processor with its lid and pulse till it becomes a frothy mixture.

Keep the processor running and open the drip hole on the lid of the processor.

Start adding the olive oil, drop by drop through the drip hole opening.

When all the olive oil is added, start adding the avocado oil in the similar manner, that is drop by drop through the drip hole opening.

Keep it blending till it becomes a smooth puree.

Finally, blend in the white pepper.

Enjoy!

Zucchini Hummus

Serving Size

Serves 18 – 20

Cooking Time

5 minutes

Nutritional Facts (Values per Serving)

Calories: 183

Total Carbohydrate: 6 g

Cholesterol: 0.5 mg

Protein: 5 g

Total Fat: 16 g

Ingredients

4 cloves of garlic, peeled and crushed

10 medium sized zucchinis, peeled and chopped

2 Tbsp ground cumin

4 Tbsp fresh lemon juice

½ cup extra virgin olive oil

4 tsp sea salt

1 ½ cup sesame tahini

½ tsp paprika

Preparation Method

Except for paprika, combine all the other ingredients in a food processor.

Pulse till all the ingredients are thoroughly blended and it becomes a smooth puree.

Take it out in a bowl or sauce container.

Garnish with paprika and serve.

Keep it refrigerated when not in use.

Paleo Style Habanero Salsa

Serving Size

Serves 8

Cooking Time

5 minutes

Nutritional Facts (Values per Serving)

Calories: 30

Total Carbohydrate: 6.7 g

Cholesterol: 0.1 mg

Protein: 1.3 g

Total Fat: 0.2 g

Ingredients

12 Italian plum tomatoes, diced

1 cup chopped red onion

2 cloves of garlic, peeled and crushed

2 Jalapeno peppers, diced

1 Habanero peppers, diced

2 Tbsp fresh lime juice

Sea salt to taste

2 cups chopped fresh cilantro

Freshly ground black pepper to taste

Preparation Method

Combine all the ingredients in a food processor.

Pulse till it becomes a smooth puree.

You can serve it with tortilla chips and Kale Krisps.

BBQ Flavored Spicy Sauce

Serving Size

Serves 16

Cooking Time

25 – 30 minutes

Nutritional Facts (Values per Serving)

Calories: 5.8

Total Carbohydrate: 6.8 g

Cholesterol: 0 mg

Protein: 1.8 g

Total Fat: 2.2 g

Ingredients

4 Tbsp apple cider vinegar

2 cups chicken stock

Half cup chopped shallot

1 ½ cup tomato paste

6 cloves of garlic, peeled and crushed

2 tsp ground cayenne pepper

2 Tbsp Dijon mustard

2 tsp ground cumin

2 tsp ground black pepper

2 tsp red pepper flakes

2 Tbsp avocado oil

2 tsp prepared horseradish

1 tsp sea salt

Preparation Method

Combine all the ingredients in a saucepan.

Bring it to a simmer over medium flame, while stirring constantly.

Reduce the heat to low.

Cover the saucepan and let it cook for 15 – 20 minutes, till the sauce attains the desired consistency while stirring after few minutes.

Roasted Red Walnut Dip

Serving Size

Makes 2 cups (about 12 servings)

Cooking Time

5 – 10 minutes

Nutritional Facts (Values per Serving)

Calories: 308

Total Carbohydrate: 8.2 g

Cholesterol: 0.0 mg

Protein: 6.5 g

Total Fat: 30 g

Ingredients

2 (12 oz.) jars of drained roasted red peppers

4 cups shelled walnuts

2 Tbsp minced garlic

4 tsp lemon juice

1 tsp salt

4 tablespoons extra virgin olive oil

1 tsp ground cumin

Preparation Method

Soak the shelled walnuts in water for 1 hour. Drain.

Combine the soaked walnuts, salt and cumin in a food processor.

Pulse till the walnuts are finely ground.

Add the remaining ingredients to the processor.

Pulse till smooth.

Take it out in a bowl and serve.

Keep it in refrigerator when not in use.

Hot and Fiery Sauce

Serving Size

Serves 18 – 20

Cooking Time

20 – 25 minutes

Nutritional Facts (Values per Serving)

Calories: 15

Total Carbohydrate: 3.4 g

Cholesterol: 0.1 mg

Protein: 0.6 g

Total Fat: 0.1 g

Ingredients

12 Italian plum tomatoes, cut in half

2 cloves of garlic

2 dried Chipotle chili peppers

2 Jalapeno peppers, seeded and chopped

2 Tbsp fresh lime juice

Half cup chopped fresh cilantro

2 small white onions, cut in quarters

Preparation Method

Fill a medium sized bowl with water and soak the chipotle peppers in it. Let sit for 15 minutes then drain.

Adjust the oven rack six inches over the heat.

Set the broiler to preheat.

Line a baking dish with aluminum foil.

Arrange tomatoes in a single layer, in the baking dish.

Put it in the oven for 12 – 15 minutes or till the skins of tomatoes are scorched.

Turn over the tomatoes and broil for 5 more minutes.

Transfer the charred tomatoes to a food processor.

Add all the remaining ingredients to the processor.

Pulse till all the ingredients are thoroughly blended and pureed.

Serve!

Paleo Main Course Recipes

Wild Salmon Delight

Serving Size

Serves 5 – 6

Cooking Time

15 minutes

Nutritional Facts (Values per Serving)

Calories: 248

Total Carbohydrate: 3 g

Cholesterol: 0.8 mg

Protein: 35 g

Total Fat: 10 g

Ingredients

2 wild salmon fillet (about 1 ½ pounds each)

2 cups finely chopped fresh basil

4 cloves of garlic, crushed

½ tsp ground black pepper

4 medium sized tomatoes, cut into thin slices

2 tsp sea salt

2 Tbsp extra virgin olive oil

Cooking spray

Preparation Method

Preheat the griller to medium heat.

Coat a double layer of aluminum foil with cooking spray.

Place the salmon fillet, skin side down, over the foil. Make sure the fillets do not touch each other.

Combine oil, salt and garlic in a bowl.

Brush this mixture over the fillets.

Spread the tomatoes evenly on both the fillets.

Finally, top it up with basil.

Grill for 12 – 15 minutes, till the fillet flakes easily.

Arrange the fillets on the serving dish.

Sprinkle the remaining basil over it and serve.

Paleo Beef with Juicy Butternut Squash

Serving Size

Serves 5 – 6

Cooking Time

6 – 8 minutes

Nutritional Facts (Values per Serving)

Calories: 337

Total Carbohydrate: 27 g

Cholesterol: 100 mg

Protein: 36 g

Total Fat: 11.3 g

Ingredients

2 cans of diced tomatoes (14 ½ oz. each)

2 pounds beef roast, cut into 1-inch cubes

1 tsp ground ginger

2 pounds butternut squash, peeled and cut into cubes

½ tsp crushed red pepper flakes

1 tsp kosher salt

1 tsp ground cumin

2 Tbsp extra virgin olive oil (substitute: coconut oil)

2 tsp paprika

1 tsp ground cinnamon

1 tsp ground turmeric

1 medium sized yellow onion, diced

½ tsp freshly ground black pepper

5 cloves of garlic, minced

Half cup chopped fresh cilantro

Preparation Method

Except for squash and cilantro, combine all the other ingredients in a slow cooker.

Mix thoroughly. Make sure the beef roast cubes are thoroughly coated.

Cover the cooker and let it cook on low heat for 5 – 6 hours, or till the meat is tender.

Stir in the squash cubes.

Cover the cooker again and cook for another 90 minutes, till the squash is soft.

Take it out in the serving dish.

Garnish with fresh cilantro and serve!

Spaghetti Squash with Veggie Fry

Serving Size

Serves 6 – 8

Cooking Time

40 – 45 minutes

Nutritional Facts (Values per Serving)

Calories: 388

Total Carbohydrate: 14.5 g

Cholesterol: 52 mg

Protein: 17 g

Total Fat: 30 g

Ingredients

1 ½ pounds ground beef

1 spaghetti squash, cut into half and remove the seeds

1 Tbsp red pepper flakes

1 zucchini, chopped

¼ cup fresh oregano, chopped

1 cup sliced mushrooms

¼ cup fresh basil, chopped

22 oz. crushed tomatoes (canned)

1 medium sized white onion, diced

1 red bell pepper, diced

1 green bell pepper, chopped

¼ cup water

1 Tbsp extra virgin olive oil

¼ cup fresh thyme, chopped

Preparation Method

Set the oven to preheat at 400°F.

Fill a baking dish with water and put the squash halves in it.

Bake the squash for 30 – 40 minutes, till the squash is tender enough to shred.

Meanwhile, place a nonstick skillet over medium-high flame.

Combine beef and onion in it. Cook till the meat is lightly browned and crumbled. Remove the skillet off the heat.

Place another nonstick skillet over medium flame and heat oil in it.

When the oil is hot, add mushrooms, zucchini, green and red bell peppers to it.

Sauté till the veggies are tender yet crispy.

Stir in the oregano, thyme, basil and crushed tomatoes.

Let it simmer for over medium flame for 10 minutes.

Now stir in the cooked beef-onion in it. Stir well.

Reduce the flame to low and cook for a few more minutes while stirring occasionally.

When the squash is tender, take it out off the oven.

Shred the squash using two forks.

Stir it in the meat-veggie skillet. Mix well.

Take it out in the serving dish.

Serve it hot!

Pork Lime Strips

Serving Size

Serves 8

Cooking Time

20 – 30 minutes

Nutritional Facts (Values per Serving)

Calories: 308

Total Carbohydrate: 14.4 g

Cholesterol: 63 mg

Protein: 22 g

Total Fat: 18 g

Ingredients

4 medium sized onions, cut into thin slices

2 pounds pork tenderloin, cut into thin slices

2 red bell peppers, thinly sliced

8 clove of garlic cloves, chopped

2 Tbsp fresh lime juice

Half extra virgin olive oil

1 cup finely chopped fresh cilantro

4 Tbsp olive pomace oil, divided

2 Tbsp chopped ginger

Preparation Method

Combine the cilantro, extra virgin olive oil, ginger and garlic in a large bowl. Mix well.

Toss the pork strips in it. Turn to coat. Let it marinade for at least one hour.

Place a nonstick skillet over medium-high flame. Heat 2 Tbsp of olive pomace oil in it.

When the oil is hot, add the pork to it.

Cook till the pork is brown and cooked through.

Take another skillet and heat the remaining olive pomace oil in it.

When the oil is hot, add onion slices to it.

Sauté till the onion is translucent.

Add the bell pepper. Sauté for 4 more minutes.

Stir in the cooked pork. Cook for 2 more minutes while stirring constantly.

Finally, stir in lime juice. Cook and stir for another minute.

Serve it hot!

Taco Stuffed Peppers

Serving Size

Serves 3 – 4

Cooking Time

35 – 45 minutes

Nutritional Facts (Values per Serving)

Calories: 587

Total Carbohydrate: 41 g

Cholesterol: 74 mg

Protein: 31 g

Total Fat: 37 g

Ingredients

4 yellow bell peppers

1 pound lean ground beef

6 oz. tomato paste

4 oz. black olives, sliced

1 large sized onion, diced

Half cup chopped fresh cilantro

3 ripe avocados, pitted and peeled

1 (1 ¼ oz.) packet of taco seasoning

1 (10 oz.) can of tomatoes with green chilies

1 tsp garlic powder

Cooking spray

Preparation Method

Set the oven to preheat at 350ºF.

Coat a baking dish with cooking spray.

Season the beef with taco seasoning.

Brown the seasoned beef in a skillet.

When the beef is browned, add onions and cilantro to it.

Sauté for 5 minutes.

Cut the bell peppers in half and remove the seeds.

Taka one half of the pepper and dice in finely.

Add the diced pepper to the beef mixture along with the canned tomatoes, olives and tomato paste. Stir to mix.

Place the remaining halves of the peppers open side up in the pan.

Spoon equal amount of the beef mixture into each pepper

Put it in the oven for 30 minutes.

Meanwhile, combine the garlic powder and avocados in a bowl.

Mash the avocados with a potato masher. Stir to mix.

When the peppers are baked, take them out in the serving plates.

Top up each pepper with a spoonful of mashed avocado mixture.

Enjoy the Paleo taco stuffed peppers!

Shrimp and Chicken Jambalaya

Serving Size

Serves 5 – 6

Cooking Time

35 – 45 minutes

Nutritional Facts (Values per Serving)

Calories: 260

Total Carbohydrate: 14.5 g

Cholesterol: 167 mg

Protein: 32 g

Total Fat: 8.5 g

Ingredients

1 cup chicken broth

1 pound shrimps (peeled, deveined and cooked)

1 Tbsp extra virgin olive oil

6 cloves of garlic, chopped

1 pound chicken breast, cooked and chopped

2 andouille sausage, cut into ¼ inch chunks

2 zucchinis, diced

1 tsp hot sauce

1 Tbsp Paleo friendly butter

1 can (14 oz.) of crushed tomatoes

3 green bell peppers, remove the seeds and chop the peppers

1 large sized onion, diced

2 Tbsp Cajun seasoning

Preparation Method

Combine the oil and butter in a saucepan. Heat over medium flame.

When the oil is hot, add the onions and andouille sausage to it.

Cook and stir till the sausage is brown.

Stir in the garlic. Sauté for 2 more minutes.

Stir in the Cajun seasoning, crushed tomatoes, chopped bell peppers, chicken broth, zucchinis and hot sauce.

Bring it to a boil then reduce the heat to simmer.

Cook for about 15 minutes or till the gravy starts to thicken.

Lastly, stir in the chicken and shrimps. Cook and stir for 3 more minutes.

Serve it hot!

Cheesy Bacon Rolls

Serving Size

Serves 7 – 8

Cooking Time

35 – 40 minutes

Nutritional Facts (Values per Serving)

Calories: 637

Total Carbohydrate: 7.4 g

Cholesterol: 93 mg

Protein: 36.8 g

Total Fat: 53 g

Ingredients

16 oz. blue cheese, crumbled

4 chicken breasts (skinless and boneless), cut the breasts into horizontal halves

12 oz. walnuts, break the walnuts into halves

16 slices of bacon

Preparation Method

Set the oven to preheat at 350°F.

Using a meat mallet, flatten the chicken breast halves.

Spoon equal amount of cheese and walnuts in the middle of each chicken slice.

Roll over the chicken slice.

Roll a slice of bacon over each chicken roll.

Insert a toothpick in the center of each roll, to keep it secured.

Place a nonstick skillet over medium flame.

Place the rolls in it and cook till the bacon is brown, about 5 minutes.

Transfer the rolls to a baking sheet.

Put it in the oven for 30 – 35 minutes, until the chicken is well cooked.

The scrumptious cheesy bacon rolls are ready to devour!

Spicy Pork Chops with Grilled Vegetables

Serving Size

Serves 8

Cooking Time

10 – 15 minutes

Nutritional Facts (Values per Serving)

Calories: 304

Total Carbohydrate: 7 g

Cholesterol: 67 mg

Protein: 29 g

Total Fat: 17 g

Ingredients

8 bone-in pork chops (about ¾ inch thick), trimmed

6 Tbsp rice vinegar

8 tsp chili powder, divided

2 tsp fish sauce

2 tsp olive oil, divided

4 tsp sugar

8 scallions, cut into thin slices

12 cups thinly sliced napa cabbage

4 Tbsp canola oil,

6 cloves of garlic, minced, divided

8 radishes, cut into small strips

1 tsp kosher salt

Preparation Method

Set the griller to preheat medium.

Grease the grill.

Take a large bowl and combine vinegar, canola oil, 2 minced cloves, sugar, 4 tsp chili powder and fish sauce. Whisk till the sugar is completely dissolved.

Stir in the radishes, cabbage and scallions. Mix well and set aside.

Take another bowl and combine the remaining minced garlic, salt and the remaining chili powder in it. Mix well.

Stir in the olive oil.

Coat both sides of the chops with chili-garlic mixture.

Grill the chops for about 5 minutes per side or till the chops are cooked through. Flip over the chops once in between.

Serve the grilled chops over the vegetable mixture.

Enjoy the succulent Spicy Pork Chops with Grilled Vegetables!

Paleo Friendly Cheesy Beef Pizza

Serving Size

Makes 1 large pizza (4 – 6 serving)

Cooking Time

15 – 20 minutes

Nutritional Facts (Values per Serving)

Calories: 506

Total Carbohydrate: 5 g

Cholesterol: 229 mg

Protein: 56.5 g

Total Fat: 27.8 g

Ingredients

3 ½ oz. packaged sliced pepperoni

2 pounds lean ground beef

Half cup Parmesan cheese, grated

1 tsp ground black pepper

Half cup mozzarella cheese, grated, divided

1 tsp garlic salt

1 cup tomato sauce

1 Tbsp sea salt

1 tsp caraway seeds

1 tsp red pepper flakes

2 free range eggs

1 tsp dried oregano

2 free range eggs

Cooking spray, of any vegetable oil

Preparation Method

Set the oven to preheat at 450oF.

Grease a pizza pan with cooking spray.

Now take a small bowl and combine the oregano, salt, garlic salt, caraway seeds, black pepper and red pepper flakes. Mix well and set aside.

Take another large bowl and combine the eggs and beef in it. Mix well.

Stir in the spice mixture and parmesan cheese.

Press an even layer of the beef mixture in the base of the greased pizza pan.

Bake for 10 minutes, till the beef is no longer pink.

Take the pan out of the oven.

Turn on the oven's broiler.

Spread one-third of the mozzarella cheese over the baked beef.

Top it up with an even layer of the tomato sauce.

Sprinkle another one-third of the mozzarella cheese.

Spread the pepperoni slices over the cheese.

Lastly, sprinkle the remaining mozzarella cheese.

Broil for 4 – 5 minutes, till the cheese melts and is lightly browned.

Slice the pizza using the pizza cutter.

Serve it hot!

Spicy Turkey Meatballs

Serving Size

Serves 8

Cooking Time

20 – 25 minutes

Nutritional Facts (Values per Serving)

Calories: 263

Total Carbohydrate: 4.6 g

Cholesterol: 125 mg

Protein: 27 g

Total Fat: 16 g

Ingredients

2 pounds ground turkey

2 tsp garlic powder

3 tsp dried oregano

2 tsp onion powder

2 free range egg

3 tsp dried parsley

1 tsp red pepper flakes

½ tsp sea salt

1 cup almond meal, divided

4 tsp dried parsley

1 tsp freshly ground black pepper

Preparation Method

Set the oven to preheat at 400°F.

Expect for the last three ingredients, combine all the other ingredients in a large bowl. Mix well.

Add half of the almond meal to it. Use your hands to mix the meat mixture and form meatballs from it (about 2½ inches diameter per meatball).

Take another bowl and combine the dried parsley, black pepper and the remaining almond meal in it.

Roll all the meatballs in the parsley-pepper mixture.

Place all the meatballs onto a cookie sheet.

Bake for 20 – 25 minutes, till the beef is browned and cooked through.

The hot and spicy turkey meatballs are ready to be served!

Lemon Shrimp Delight

Serving Size

Makes 12 shrimps

Cooking Time

15 – 20 minutes

Nutritional Facts (Values per Serving)

Calories: 388

Total Carbohydrate: 5.8 g

Cholesterol: 192 mg

Protein: 21 g

Total Fat: 31.7 g

Ingredients

12 large shrimps, peeled and deveined

½ Tbsp lemon zest

¼ cup fresh lemon juice

2 cloves of garlic, crushed

¼ cup extra virgin olive oil

Half medium onion, finely chopped

½ Tbsp coconut oil

½ Tbsp grated ginger

½ tsp ground turmeric

Preparation Method

Take a bowl and add in it the lemon juice, extra virgin olive oil, the lemon zest, onion, ginger, ground turmeric and garlic. Mix well.

Toss the shrimps. Turn to coat.

Plastic wrap the bowl and put it in the refrigerator to marinade for 2 hours at least.

Place a nonstick skillet over medium-high flame and heat the coconut oil in it.

When the oil is hot, add the shrimps to it. Do not put its marinade yet.

Stir and cook for about 10 minutes, till the shrimps are pink.

Stir in the marinade.

Bring it to a boil while stirring constantly.

Serve it hot!

Almond Tuna Patties

Serving Size

Makes 8 burger patties

Cooking Time

10 minutes per patty

Nutritional Facts (Values per Serving)

Calories: 340

Total Carbohydrate: 6 g

Cholesterol: 193 mg

Protein: 39.8 g

Total Fat: 17.4 g

Ingredients

19 oz. canned tuna, drained

6 free range eggs

Half cup fresh chopped cilantro

4 Tbsp Balsamic vinegar

1 cup almond meal

4 Tbsp fresh lemon juice

Sea salt to taste

4 Tbsp extra virgin olive oil

2 Tbsp grated ginger root

Freshly ground black pepper to taste

Olive oil for frying (about 2 Tbsp)

Preparation Method

Put the tuna in a large bowl along with balsamic vinegar, cilantro, ginger, extra virgin olive oil, salt, lemon juice, black pepper, almond meal and eggs. Mix well.

Divide the mixture equally into 8 equal parts and form a burger patty of each part.

Place a nonstick skillet over medium flame and heat 2 Tbsp olive oil in it.

Fry the burger patties in it for about 5 minutes per side, till it is browned and crispy. If your skillet is small, fry in batches using a little olive oil for every patty.

Serve with any of your favorite dip.

Paleo Dessert Recipes

Avocado Chocolate Mousse

Serving Size

Serves 8

Cooking Time

5 minutes (4 – 5 hours refrigeration)

Nutritional Facts (Values per Serving)

Calories: 276

Total Carbohydrate: 41 g

Cholesterol: 0.1 mg

Protein: 2.5 g

Total Fat: 14 g

Ingredients

240 ml thick coconut milk (about 1 cup)

1 tsp vanilla extract

2 ripe avocados, peeled, pitted and coarsely diced

2 Tbsp arrowroot

Half cup cocoa powder (unsweetened)

6 Tbsp honey

Chopped walnuts, to garnish

Preparation Method

Except for walnuts, combine all the other ingredients in a food processor.

Pulse till it becomes a smooth mixture.

Pour it into desert bowls.

Garnish with walnuts.

Refrigerate for 4 – 5 hours.

The delicious Avocado Chocolate Mousse Loaf is ready to devour!

Apple and Pear Cake with Honey Walnut Topping

Serving Size

Makes 1 cake (about 8 servings)

Cooking Time

50 – 60 minutes

Nutritional Facts (Values per Serving)

Calories: 528

Total Carbohydrate: 48 g

Cholesterol: 178 mg

Protein: 10 g

Total Fat: 35.4 g

Ingredients for Cake

2 tsp fresh lemon juice

1 medium apple, cored, peeled and cut into thin slices

¼ cup arrowroot powder

½ tsp baking soda

5 free range eggs

¼ cup raw honey

¾ cup coconut milk

2 pears, cored, peeled and cut into thin slices

¾ tsp baking powder

4 oz. grass fed butter

1 tsp vanilla essence

¾ cup coconut flour

½ tsp sea salt

Cooking spray, of coconut oil

Ingredients for Honey Walnut Topping

1 tsp ground cinnamon

2 Tbsp coconut flour

2 oz. grass fed butter, cut into 1 inch cubes

3 Tbsp raw honey

¾ cup chopped walnuts

Preparation Method

Set the oven to preheat at 350°F.

Take a spring form pan and wrap the base of it with aluminum foil.

Coat the insides of the pan with cooking spray.

Take a bowl and add in it the walnuts, ground cinnamon and 3 Tbsp raw honey. Mix well.

Take another bowl and combine the butter cubes and 2 Tbsp coconut flour in it. Mix till it becomes crumbly.

Stir in the honey-walnut mixture. Mix well and set aside.

Now take another bowl and combine the apples, lemon juice and pear in it. Mix well and set aside.

Take another large bowl and add in the half cup softened butter, ¼ cup raw honey and free range eggs. Beat well using an electric beater.

Stir in the arrowroot powder, coconut milk, vanilla essence, baking powder, coconut flour, baking soda, and sea salt. Whisk well.

Transfer half of this batter into the prepared springform pan.

Pour the apple-pear mixture evenly over it.

Pour in the remaining batter.

Spread the walnut mixture over it.

Bake for about 50 minutes, or till a cake tested when inserted into the center of the cake comes out clean.

Allow it to cool in the pan for 10 minutes.

Take it out in the rack or serving plate and let it cool for 60 more minutes.

Enjoy!

Zesty Date Tarts

Serving Size

Makes 8 tarts

Cooking Time

10 – 15 minutes

Nutritional Facts (Values per Tart)

Calories: 244

Total Carbohydrate: 20 g

Cholesterol: 106 mg

Protein: 9.5 g

Total Fat: 16.5 g

Ingredients for Crust

2 cup almond meal

6 Tbsp fresh lemon juice

8 dates, pitted

Ingredients for Filling

12 Tbsp fresh lemon juice

4 tsp lemon zest

4 free range eggs, beaten

2 Tbsp raw honey

Preparation Method

Set oven to preheat at 350°F.

Put paper liners in 4 muffin tins.

Combine all the curst ingredients in a food processor.

Pulse till all the ingredients are thoroughly mixed.

Divide the mixture equally into 8 parts.

Press each part of the crust evenly and firmly into the base and up the sides of the muffin paper liners.

Bake for 10 minutes, till the crust is golden brown.

Meanwhile, prepare the tart filling.

To make the tart filling,

Place a saucepan over low heat. Add in the lemon zest, lemon juice and honey.

Bring it to simmer.

Start adding the beaten eggs slowly and gradually in to the saucepan, while whisking fast and constantly.

When all the eggs are thoroughly whisked in the saucepan, turn off the heat.

Allow it cool for 5 minutes.

Spoon equal amount of filling in each crust.

Refrigerate the tarts for at max 20 minutes.

Enjoy!

Chocolicious Banana Cinnamon Loaf

Serving Size

Serves 8

Cooking Time

50 minutes

Nutritional Facts (Values per Serving)

Calories: 355

Total Carbohydrate: 35.6 g

Cholesterol: 110 mg

Protein: 9 g

Total Fat: 23 g

Ingredients

Half cup coconut flour

4 free range eggs

1 tsp baking soda

1 tsp coconut oil

Half cup almond butter

1 Tbsp grass fed butter, softened

1 cup chocolate chips (semi sweet)

1 cup mashed bananas

1 Tbsp ground cinnamon

Cooking spray, of coconut oil

Pinch of kosher salt

Preparation Method

Set oven to preheat at 350°F.

Coat the insides of a 9 x 5 inches loaf pan with cooking spray.

Combine the butter, coconut oil and chocolate chips in a microwave safe bowl.

Cover the bowl and microwave till all the three ingredients are melted.

Stir in the ground cinnamon.

Take another large bowl and mix the baking soda, coconut flour, and kosher salt in it. Mix well.

Fold the flour mixture into the mashes bananas.

Now take another bowl and combine the free range eggs and almond butter in it.

Beat using an electric beater, till it is smooth and creamy.

Pour this mixture into the mashed banana mixture. Mix well.

Transfer half of this batter into the greased loaf pan.

Spread half of the melted chocolate mixture evenly over the batter.

Pour the remaining batter over the chocolate mixture in the loaf pan.

Finally, top it up with the remaining chocolate mixture.

Bake the loaf for about 50 minutes or till cooked through.

Allow it to cool for 10 minutes.

The delectable Chocolicious Banana Cinnamon Loaf is ready to serve!

Paleo Style Pumpkin Vanilla Custard

Serving Size

Serves 6

Cooking Time

45 minutes

Nutritional Facts (Values per Serving)

Calories: 129

Total Carbohydrate: 24 g

Cholesterol: 1.3 mg

Protein: 3.7 g

Total Fat: 0.2 g

Ingredients

1 ½ cup cooked pumpkin

½ tsp vanilla extract

4 egg whites of free range eggs

1 tsp ground cinnamon

1 ½ almond milk

½ tsp ginger

½ cup sugar

Preparation Method

Set oven to preheat at 350°F.

Combine all the ingredients in a bowl.

Divide the mixture equally into 6 custard bowls or ramekins.

Put it in the preheated oven for about 45 minutes, or till a toothpick when inserted in the center comes out clean.

Allow it to cool for a while.

Tastes best when chilled!

Cranberry and Nut Protein Bars

Serving Size

Makes 18 – 20 protein bars

Cooking Time

70 – 80 minutes

Nutritional Facts (Values per Serving)

Calories: 356

Total Carbohydrate: 25 g

Cholesterol: 0.2 mg

Protein: 12.5 g

Total Fat: 25 g

Ingredients

1 cup chopped pecans

1 ½ tsp ground cinnamon

¼ cup raw honey

1 cup vanilla flavored protein powder

1 Tbsp vanilla essence

1 ½ tsp molasses

1 cup pumpkin seeds

Half cup raisins

Half cup pitted dates

2 cups sliced almonds

Half cup coconut flour

2 cups chopped walnuts

1 cup dried cranberries

3 Tbsp coconut oil

Cooking spray

Preparation Method

Set oven to preheat at 220°F.

Combine the walnuts and pecans in a bowl and then spread them evenly in the base of a nonstick baking pan.

Put the pan in the preheated oven for about 30 minutes, till the walnuts and pecans are roasted,

Transfer the roasted nuts to a plate. Set aside.

Now increase the temperature of oven to 230oF.

Grease a 9 x 13 inches baking dish with cooking spray.

Combine the almonds, roasted walnuts and pecan in a food processor.

Pulse till all the three nuts are coarsely chopped.

Transfer it to a bowl.

Add the cranberries, coconut oil, pumpkin seeds, pitted dates, raw honey, protein powder, raisins, cinnamon powder, coconut flour, molasses and vanilla essence to the chopped nuts. Mix well.

Press this mixture evenly in to the base of the prepared baking dish.

Put the dish in the preheated oven for about 40 minutes, till golden brown.

Allow it to cool for 10 minutes.

Cut it into bars and serve!

Keep the protein bars in an airtight container when not in use.

Applesauce Muffins with Raspberry Topping

Serving Size

Makes 12 muffins

Cooking Time

25 – 30 minutes

Nutritional Facts (Values per Serving)

Calories: 197

Total Carbohydrate: 22 g

Cholesterol: 53 mg

Protein: 2 g

Total Fat: 11.6 g

Ingredients

3 free range eggs

Half cup applesauce

¼ tsp baking soda

Half cup coconut oil, melted

Half cup coconut flour

3 Tbsp honey

½ tsp sea salt

Half cup raspberry jam

1 Tbsp almond milk

3 Tbsp vanilla essence

Preparation Method

Set oven to preheat at 350°F.

Line 12 muffin tins with paper liners.

Combine the free range eggs, applesauce, honey, coconut oil and vanilla essence in a food processor.

Pulse till all the ingredients are thoroughly mixed.

Transfer it to a large bowl.

Stir in the sea salt, baking soda and coconut flour. Mix well.

Add almond milk to it. Mix well.

Spoon the batter in the paper lined muffin tins, while filling 2/3 of each tin.

Swirl a spoonful raspberry jam over each muffin.

Bake for about 25 minutes or till a toothpick when inserted in the middle of the cupcake comes out clean.

Enjoy!

Frozen Fruit Delight

Serving Size

Makes 12 pieces (about 6 servings)

Cooking Time

5 minutes plus 60 minutes refrigeration

Nutritional Facts (Values per Serving)

Calories: 45

Total Carbohydrate: 10.6 g

Cholesterol: 1 mg

Protein: 0.9 g

Total Fat: 0.3 g

Ingredients

4 ripe bananas

2/3 cup peeled and coarsely diced oranges

Half cup almond milk

Preparation Method

Line 12 cupcake cups with paper liners.

Mash the bananas.

Combine the mashed bananas and milk in a bowl.

Fold in the chopped oranges.

Spoon equal amount of this mixture into each paper lined cupcake

Freeze for 60 minutes, till it becomes solid.

Take it out of the freezer and allow it to defrost just 10 minutes before serving.

Enjoy!

Banana Coconut Waffles

Serving Size

Serves 8

Cooking Time

25 – 30 minutes

Nutritional Facts (Values per Serving)

Calories: 333

Total Carbohydrate: 34.5 g

Cholesterol: 108 mg

Protein: 10.5 g

Total Fat: 18.4 g

Ingredients

1 cup mashed ripe banana

1 cup shredded coconut (unsweetened)

¼ tsp baking soda

1 tsp ground cinnamon

Half cup whey protein powder

¼ tsp sea salt

4 Tbsp dark maple syrup

1 cup almond flour

¼ tsp baking powder

Half cup milk

3 tsp vanilla extract

4 egg yolks

6 egg whites

Preparation Method

Grease a waffle iron and then set it to preheat, according to the manufacturer's instructions.

Put the coconut in a food processor. Pulse for a few times, till the coconut is finely powdered

Transfer it to a large bowl.

Stir in the almond flour, baking soda, sea salt, baking powder, ground cinnamon and whey protein powder. Set aside.

In another small bowl, combine the milk, mashes bananas, maple syrup and vanilla extract.

Stir in the egg yolks. Whisk well.

Beat the egg whites using an electric beater, till it becomes stiff and foamy. Remove the beater and whisk manually till it forms sharp peaks.

Fold the banana mixture into the whey protein powder mixture. Mix well.

Stir in 1/3 of the beaten egg whites. Mix well.

Fold in the remaining egg whites.

Scoop the batter into the preheated iron, according to the measurements recommended by the manufacturer.

Cook till the waffle is golden and crispy, 3 – 5 minutes.

Repeat the same with the remaining batter.

Serve it hot and crispy.

To make it more delectable and filling, top up each waffle with a scoop of your favorite ice cream.